UNDERSTANDING

RESVERATROL

AND BENEFITS

A Guide To Knowing Its Major Targets, Scientific Focus Areas, And Key Health Advantages

DR. LACEY MICHELLE

Disclaimer:

The information provided in this book is for general informational purposes only and is not intended as medical advice.

Readers are encouraged to consult with a qualified healthcare professional for any health concerns or questions.

The author of this book is not affiliated with any individual, website, organization, or products mentioned within.

This book does not endorse or promote any specific brands, services, or external entities. Any references made are purely for illustrative purposes and should not be construed as endorsements.

Readers are responsible for their own decisions and should conduct their own research before making any health-related choices.

Any liability resulting from the use of this information, whether direct or indirect, is disclaimed by the author and publisher.

Contents

About The Book

CHAPTER ONE

What Is Resveratrol?

Resveratrol is a natural polyphenolic compound that has gained significant attention in the world of science and health due to its potential benefits for human well-being.

This compound is part of a group of phytochemicals known as stilbenes and is primarily found in various plant species. One of the most well-known sources of resveratrol is red wine, which has led to considerable interest and research into its potential health effects.

Resveratrol is known for its antioxidant properties and has been investigated for its potential role in promoting longevity and preventing various chronic diseases, such as heart disease and cancer.

The Origins Of Resveratrol

The origins of resveratrol can be traced back to the natural defense mechanisms of plants. It is produced by various plant species, including grapes, peanuts, and certain types of berries, as a response to environmental stressors like fungal infections and ultraviolet (UV) radiation.

When plants are exposed to such stressors, they produce resveratrol as a protective compound. Interestingly, this is where the connection to red wine comes in, as grapes, especially red grapes, contain significant amounts of resveratrol, which is extracted during the winemaking process.

Resveratrol's presence in red wine has been the subject of much research and debate, as it has been suggested that moderate consumption of red wine might contribute to the "French Paradox," which is the observation that despite a diet relatively high in saturated fats, the French population has a lower incidence of heart disease. This paradox has been attributed, at least in part, to the potential health benefits of resveratrol.

Chemical Structure And Properties
Resveratrol's chemical structure consists of two phenol rings connected by a carbon-carbon double bond, forming a distinctive trans-stilbene structure.

This structure is responsible for its biological activity and antioxidant properties.

Resveratrol exists in two main forms: trans-resveratrol and cis-resveratrol, with the trans form being more biologically active and abundant in nature.

One of the remarkable properties of resveratrol is its ability to scavenge free radicals, which are highly reactive molecules that can cause oxidative stress and damage to cells.

By neutralizing these free radicals, resveratrol can help protect cells and tissues from oxidative damage, which is associated with various chronic diseases and the aging process.

Moreover, resveratrol has been found to activate sirtuins, a family of proteins that play a key role in regulating cellular processes related to aging and metabolism.

This activation has led to considerable interest in resveratrol's potential to extend lifespan and improve overall health.

Natural Sources Of Resveratrol

Resveratrol is naturally present in a wide range of plant-based foods and beverages. As mentioned earlier, grapes, particularly the skins of red grapes, are among the most well-known sources of resveratrol.

Other natural sources of this compound include peanuts, certain types of berries, such as blueberries and cranberries, and red wine. Japanese knotweed, a plant used in traditional medicine, is also rich in resveratrol.

While red wine is often highlighted for its resveratrol content, it's essential to note that resveratrol levels can vary significantly between different wine varieties and brands. Additionally, consuming red wine in moderation is crucial, as excessive alcohol intake can have adverse health effects.

In recent years, resveratrol supplements have become increasingly popular as a means to ensure a consistent intake of this compound.

These supplements are available in various forms, such as capsules, tablets, and liquid extracts.

When considering resveratrol supplementation, it's essential to consult with a healthcare professional to determine the appropriate dosage and potential benefits based on individual health and wellness goals.

resveratrol is a natural compound with a unique chemical structure and intriguing properties.

Its origins in plant defense mechanisms, antioxidant effects, and potential health benefits have made it a subject of extensive scientific research and public interest.

While natural sources like grapes and red wine provide opportunities to incorporate resveratrol into one's diet, supplements have become a convenient option for those seeking to harness its potential benefits.

As the field of resveratrol research continues to evolve, it holds promise for improving human health and well-being.

CHAPTER TWO

Health Benefits Of Resveratrol

Antioxidant Properties:

Resveratrol, a natural polyphenol found in various plant sources, has gained significant attention for its antioxidant properties. Antioxidants play a crucial role in neutralizing harmful free radicals in the body, which can damage cells and contribute to various chronic diseases. Resveratrol's ability to scavenge free radicals helps protect cells from oxidative stress and may contribute to overall health and well-being.

Cardiovascular Health:

Resveratrol has been extensively studied for its potential benefits in promoting cardiovascular health. It is believed to enhance the function of blood vessels and reduce the risk of atherosclerosis, a condition where arteries become clogged with plaque. Moreover, resveratrol can help lower blood pressure and improve lipid profiles, which may reduce the risk of heart disease and stroke.

Anti-Inflammatory Effects:

Chronic inflammation is at the root of many diseases, including cardiovascular diseases, cancer, and neurodegenerative disorders. Resveratrol has demonstrated anti-inflammatory properties by inhibiting the production of pro-inflammatory molecules and promoting the expression of anti-inflammatory factors.

By reducing chronic inflammation, resveratrol may contribute to better overall health.

Longevity And Aging:

Resveratrol has been linked to the promotion of longevity and slowing down the aging process. Studies in various model organisms have shown that resveratrol can extend lifespan by activating certain longevity-related genes.

While the effects in humans are still being researched, the compound's potential to enhance the quality of life in later years is a subject of ongoing investigation.

Potential Cancer Benefits:

Research suggests that resveratrol may have potential cancer-fighting properties. It has been shown to inhibit the growth of cancer cells and promote apoptosis, a process that leads to the self-destruction of damaged or cancerous cells.

Resveratrol may also interfere with the development of blood vessels that support tumor growth. However, it's important to note that more research is needed to fully understand its efficacy in cancer prevention and treatment.

Neuroprotective Effects:

The brain-protective properties of resveratrol have generated considerable interest in its potential to support brain health. It can protect nerve cells from damage, reduce inflammation in the brain, and enhance cognitive function.

Studies have explored its role in potentially preventing or delaying the onset of neurodegenerative conditions such as Alzheimer's and Parkinson's disease, offering hope for improving the quality of life for those at risk.

resveratrol is a compound with a wide range of potential health benefits, primarily attributed to its antioxidant, anti-inflammatory, and cell-protective properties.

While it has shown promise in various health-related areas, it's important to acknowledge that more research is needed to fully understand the extent of its effects in humans and the optimal dosages required for specific health benefits.

Incorporating resveratrol-rich foods or supplements into a balanced diet may be a step towards reaping its potential rewards, but it should be done in consultation with healthcare professionals, especially for individuals with underlying health conditions.

CHAPTER THREE

Resveratrol And Weight Management

Resveratrol, a natural polyphenol found in various plant sources, has gained significant attention for its potential role in weight management and its impact on various aspects of metabolism.

This compound is most commonly associated with red wine and is believed to be one of the factors contributing to the "French Paradox," where despite a diet rich in saturated fats, the French population has lower rates of cardiovascular diseases.

The interest in resveratrol's potential health benefits, including its effects on weight management, has led to extensive research in recent years.

Metabolism And Weight Loss

Metabolism plays a critical role in determining an individual's ability to gain, lose, or maintain weight. Resveratrol has been studied for its ability to influence metabolism, particularly in relation to energy expenditure and fat storage.

Research suggests that resveratrol may have a positive impact on metabolism by increasing the activity of specific genes and proteins involved in fat metabolism, including SIRT1, which is a key regulator of cellular energy balance.

Moreover, resveratrol has been found to activate brown adipose tissue (BAT), which is known to increase energy expenditure by generating heat.

BAT is responsible for burning calories to maintain body temperature, making it an attractive target for weight management. By enhancing BAT activity, resveratrol may contribute to an increase in overall energy expenditure, potentially aiding in weight loss efforts.

Resveratrol And Obesity

Obesity is a global health concern, with numerous associated health risks such as diabetes, cardiovascular disease, and certain cancers. Studies have investigated the potential anti-obesity effects of resveratrol. One key mechanism involves the regulation of adipogenesis, the process by which new fat cells are formed.

Resveratrol has been shown to inhibit the differentiation of pre-adipocytes into mature fat cells, reducing the accumulation of fat in adipose tissues.

Resveratrol's impact on inflammation and insulin sensitivity also plays a significant role in combating obesity.

Chronic inflammation and insulin resistance are often linked to obesity and metabolic disorders. Resveratrol exhibits anti-inflammatory properties and can improve insulin sensitivity, potentially helping individuals manage their weight more effectively.

Role In Appetite Control

Appetite control is another essential aspect of weight management. Resveratrol has been studied for its potential to influence appetite and food intake.

Some research suggests that resveratrol may affect appetite-regulating hormones, such as leptin and ghrelin, which are involved in signaling hunger and fullness. By modulating these hormones, resveratrol could potentially help individuals make healthier food choices and consume fewer calories.

In addition to hormonal regulation, resveratrol's interaction with the gut microbiota has also been explored. The gut microbiota plays a crucial role in metabolism and appetite regulation.

Resveratrol may positively impact the gut microbiome, promoting the growth of beneficial bacteria that could aid in weight management.

while resveratrol holds promise in the realm of weight management, it's important to note that the effects may vary among individuals, and more research is needed to establish concrete recommendations for its use.

As with any dietary supplement, it is essential to consult with a healthcare professional before incorporating resveratrol into your weight management plan, especially if you have underlying medical conditions or are taking medications that could interact with the compound.

Nonetheless, the scientific exploration of resveratrol's potential benefits in metabolism, obesity prevention, and appetite control continues to provide intriguing insights into its potential role in supporting a healthy weight.

CHAPTER FOUR

Resveratrol And Skin Health

Resveratrol, a natural polyphenol found in red grapes, red wine, and some other plants, has gained significant attention for its potential benefits in promoting skin health. This antioxidant compound is known for its diverse range of properties, including its role in anti-aging, skin protection, and enhancing skin radiance.

In this discussion, we will explore the science behind resveratrol's impact on skin health and its various applications, with a specific focus on its role in anti-aging, skin protection, and topical use.

Anti-Aging Properties

One of the most prominent aspects of resveratrol's influence on skin health is its potential anti-aging properties. Resveratrol is celebrated for its ability to combat the signs of aging, including fine lines, wrinkles, and loss of skin elasticity.

This is primarily attributed to its potent antioxidant activity, which helps neutralize harmful free radicals in the skin. Free radicals can damage skin cells and accelerate the aging process, resulting in the formation of wrinkles and the breakdown of collagen and elastin, which are essential for skin's firmness and suppleness.

Resveratrol's anti-aging effects extend beyond its antioxidant properties. Studies have suggested that resveratrol may activate certain genes associated with longevity, such as the sirtuin family, particularly SIRT1.

These genes play a role in cellular repair and protection, and their activation by resveratrol can help maintain skin health and slow down the aging process. Furthermore, resveratrol's ability to stimulate collagen production and inhibit enzymes that break down collagen and elastin can contribute to firmer, more youthful-looking skin.

Skin Protection And Radiance

Resveratrol also offers significant benefits in terms of skin protection and radiance. Exposure to UV radiation from the sun is a major contributor to skin damage, including sunburn, premature aging, and skin cancer. Resveratrol's protective properties make it a valuable addition to skincare regimens.

It can act as a shield against UV-induced damage by reducing inflammation and oxidative stress in the skin, potentially reducing the risk of sunburn and skin cancer.

In addition to its protective capabilities, resveratrol can enhance skin radiance and texture.

It promotes even skin tone by inhibiting the formation of melanin, the pigment responsible for dark spots and uneven skin color.

This can help diminish the appearance of age spots and other pigment-related skin issues, leaving the skin with a more youthful and glowing appearance.

Topical Resveratrol Applications

Topical applications of resveratrol have become increasingly popular in skincare products.

These products, such as creams, serums, and lotions, are formulated to deliver resveratrol directly to the skin. When applied topically, resveratrol can be absorbed into the epidermis, the outer layer of the skin, where it exerts its protective and rejuvenating effects.

Topical resveratrol products are often combined with other beneficial ingredients, such as vitamin C and hyaluronic acid, to further enhance their efficacy.

 The synergistic action of these compounds can address a wide range of skin concerns, from hydration to UV protection and wrinkle reduction.

resveratrol has demonstrated a promising role in promoting skin health through its anti-aging, skin protection, and radiance-enhancing properties.

Whether consumed as part of a balanced diet or applied topically in skincare products, resveratrol can be a valuable addition to one's routine for maintaining healthy, youthful, and radiant skin.

However, it's important to note that individual responses to resveratrol may vary, and consulting with a healthcare professional or dermatologist is advisable before incorporating resveratrol into your skincare regimen, especially if you have specific skin conditions or concerns.

CHAPTER FIVE

Resveratrol And Diabetes

Resveratrol, a natural polyphenol found in various plants such as grapes, berries, and peanuts, has garnered significant attention in recent years for its potential health benefits. Among the many areas of interest, its connection with diabetes has been a subject of intense research.

Diabetes is a complex metabolic disorder characterized by impaired regulation of blood sugar levels, and it comes in various forms, with Type 2 diabetes being the most common.

Resveratrol's impact on diabetes primarily relates to its role in managing blood sugar, improving insulin sensitivity, and its potential for preventing or managing Type 2 diabetes.

Managing Blood Sugar

One of the key factors in diabetes management is maintaining stable blood sugar levels. Resveratrol has been studied for its ability to modulate glucose metabolism and improve glycemic control. It is thought to influence several pathways related to glucose regulation.

Research suggests that resveratrol can enhance the uptake of glucose into cells, improve the function of pancreatic beta cells responsible for insulin secretion, and reduce the production of glucose by the liver. These effects collectively contribute to better blood sugar management.

Furthermore, resveratrol may help reduce the post-meal spike in blood sugar levels, which is particularly important for individuals with diabetes. It is believed to do this by inhibiting the enzymes responsible for breaking down carbohydrates in the gut, thus slowing down the absorption of sugars and promoting a more gradual increase in blood glucose after meals.

This property of resveratrol can be especially beneficial for those who need to regulate their blood sugar levels, including individuals with prediabetes or Type 2 diabetes.

Insulin Sensitivity

Another critical aspect of diabetes is insulin sensitivity, or the body's responsiveness to insulin, a hormone that plays a central role in regulating blood sugar.

In insulin-resistant conditions like Type 2 diabetes, the body's cells become less sensitive to insulin's actions, leading to elevated blood sugar levels.

Resveratrol has shown promise in enhancing insulin sensitivity, which is a key factor in preventing and managing diabetes.

Studies have demonstrated that resveratrol can activate certain signaling pathways that improve insulin sensitivity.

It is believed to increase the translocation of glucose transporters (GLUT4) to the cell membrane, making it easier for cells to take up glucose in response to insulin.

Improved insulin sensitivity not only helps lower blood sugar levels but also reduces the burden on the pancreas, as it requires less insulin to achieve the same glucose-lowering effect.

Potential For Type 2 Diabetes

Type 2 diabetes is a major health concern worldwide, and finding effective strategies for its prevention and management is essential. Resveratrol's potential in this regard is intriguing.

While it's not a cure for diabetes, the scientific evidence suggests that resveratrol supplementation, in combination with a healthy lifestyle, may reduce the risk of developing Type 2 diabetes and aid in its management.

Several epidemiological studies have observed a lower prevalence of Type 2 diabetes among individuals who consume a diet rich in foods containing resveratrol, such as red wine and grapes.

While these studies are promising, more rigorous clinical trials are needed to confirm these findings and establish the optimal dosage of resveratrol for diabetes prevention.

resveratrol holds promise in the realm of diabetes management and prevention. Its potential to manage blood sugar, improve insulin sensitivity, and reduce the risk of Type 2 diabetes has made it an attractive subject of scientific investigation.

However, it's essential to consult with a healthcare professional before incorporating resveratrol supplements into your diabetes management plan, as individual responses may vary, and its effectiveness as an adjunct therapy to standard diabetes treatments should be carefully evaluated.

CHAPTER SIX

Resveratrol And Exercise Performance

Resveratrol, a natural polyphenol found in certain foods, particularly in red grapes and red wine, has garnered significant attention in recent years for its potential health benefits.

One intriguing area of research is its impact on exercise performance. This compound has demonstrated a range of physiological effects that are relevant to athletes and individuals looking to improve their exercise capacity.

In this discussion, we will delve into the influence of resveratrol on three key aspects of exercise performance: muscle endurance, mitochondrial function, and overall athletic performance.

Muscle Endurance

Muscle endurance is a critical factor in any form of exercise, be it endurance sports, weightlifting, or cardiovascular training. Several studies have explored the role of resveratrol in enhancing muscle endurance.

Resveratrol's ability to activate the SIRT1 protein, which is involved in regulating cellular energy production, has been of particular interest.

It is thought that SIRT1 activation by resveratrol can lead to improved muscle performance by increasing the efficiency of energy utilization and reducing fatigue.

However, the evidence in this area is still inconclusive, with some studies reporting positive effects on muscle endurance, while others do not show significant benefits. Further research is needed to clarify the precise mechanisms and conditions under which resveratrol might improve muscle endurance.

Mitochondrial Function

Mitochondria, often referred to as the "powerhouses" of cells, play a central role in energy production and are vital for exercise performance.

Resveratrol has been shown to promote mitochondrial function by enhancing biogenesis (the creation of new mitochondria) and improving mitochondrial quality.

This is particularly important for endurance athletes who rely heavily on mitochondrial energy production during prolonged exercise. By bolstering mitochondrial function, resveratrol may help individuals sustain higher energy levels, delay fatigue, and improve their overall exercise performance. However, the dosage and duration of resveratrol supplementation needed to achieve these effects remain topics of ongoing research.

Athletic Performance

The overall impact of resveratrol on athletic performance is a complex and multifaceted subject.

While there is growing interest in the potential benefits of resveratrol, especially for endurance athletes, it is essential to consider the broader context of an individual's training, diet, and genetic factors.

Some studies have suggested that resveratrol may enhance cardiovascular health, which can indirectly improve athletic performance by supporting better blood circulation and oxygen delivery to muscles.

Additionally, resveratrol's anti-inflammatory and antioxidant properties may aid in post-exercise recovery and injury prevention.

However, it is important to note that the effects of resveratrol can vary from person to person, and more research is needed to establish clear guidelines for its use in athletic settings.

resveratrol's potential influence on exercise performance is a promising area of research. While it has shown promise in enhancing muscle endurance, improving mitochondrial function, and potentially benefiting athletic performance, the results are not yet definitive.

Athletes and individuals considering resveratrol supplementation should consult with healthcare professionals and be mindful of the current limitations in our understanding of how this compound interacts with various exercise regimens and individual factors.

As the research on resveratrol continues to evolve, a clearer picture of its benefits and optimal usage for exercise performance will likely emerge.

CHAPTER SEVEN

Resveratrol Supplements

Resveratrol is a natural compound found in certain foods, particularly in red grapes, red wine, and berries.

It has gained significant attention in recent years due to its potential health benefits, particularly its antioxidant properties and its association with anti-aging effects.

While resveratrol can be obtained through dietary sources, many individuals opt for resveratrol supplements to ensure they are getting a consistent and concentrated dose of this compound.

In this discussion, we will delve into various aspects of resveratrol supplements, including choosing the right supplement, dosage and usage guidelines, and potential side effects and interactions.

Choosing The Right Supplement

When it comes to choosing a resveratrol supplement, several factors need to be considered. The first step is to select a reputable brand or manufacturer.

Quality and purity vary among supplements, so it's crucial to do thorough research and choose a brand with a good track record and positive customer reviews.

Look for supplements that use high-quality, standardized resveratrol extract, as this ensures a consistent and known concentration of the compound.

Another important factor is the form of resveratrol used in the supplement. There are two primary forms: trans-resveratrol and cis-resveratrol.

Trans-resveratrol is the more biologically active form and is generally preferred in supplements.

Additionally, some resveratrol supplements may include other beneficial compounds, such as quercetin or grape seed extract, which can enhance its effects.

Consider your specific health goals and consult with a healthcare professional to determine which supplement is most appropriate for your needs.

Dosage And Usage Guidelines
Determining the right dosage of resveratrol can be a complex task, as it depends on various factors, including age, weight, and overall health.

Generally, resveratrol supplements come in a range of dosages, typically between 100 mg and 500 mg per serving. It's advisable to start with a lower dose and gradually increase it while monitoring for any adverse effects.

Resveratrol supplements are often taken with a meal to enhance absorption.

This is because resveratrol is fat-soluble, meaning it is better absorbed in the presence of dietary fats.

However, the specific timing and frequency of dosing may vary depending on the product's instructions or your healthcare provider's recommendations.

It's crucial to emphasize that resveratrol supplements are not a one-size-fits-all solution.

Individual responses to resveratrol can vary, and what works for one person may not be suitable for another.

Consulting a healthcare professional is advisable to determine the optimal dosage and usage for your unique circumstances.

Potential Side Effects And Interactions
While resveratrol is generally considered safe when used as directed, it can have potential side effects and interactions, especially at higher doses.

Some common side effects include digestive issues such as diarrhea, nausea, or stomach cramps. These side effects can often be mitigated by taking the supplement with food.

Resveratrol may also interact with certain medications, particularly blood thinners like warfarin or antiplatelet drugs.

It has mild blood-thinning properties of its own, so combining it with these medications may increase the risk of bleeding. If you are taking any medications, especially those with potential interactions, consult your healthcare provider before starting a resveratrol supplement.

resveratrol supplements can be a valuable addition to one's health regimen, thanks to their potential antioxidant and anti-aging properties.

However, it's essential to choose a high-quality supplement, follow appropriate dosage and usage guidelines, and be aware of potential side effects and interactions.

Always consult with a healthcare professional before starting any new supplement, especially if you have underlying medical conditions or are taking medications.

With proper care and guidance, resveratrol supplements can be a valuable tool in promoting overall well-being.

CHAPTER EIGHT

Food Sources Of Resveratrol

Resveratrol, a naturally occurring polyphenol, has garnered considerable attention in recent years due to its potential health benefits.

It is found in a variety of food sources, with red wine being one of the most well-known reservoirs.

However, there are several other dietary sources of resveratrol, and understanding where to find this compound can help individuals make informed choices regarding their diet and potential supplementation.

Red Wine And Resveratrol

Red wine has long been associated with resveratrol, and it is often touted as a source of this beneficial compound.

Resveratrol is primarily found in the skin of red grapes, which is why red wine contains more resveratrol than white wine.

 The fermentation process of red wine allows the extraction of resveratrol from grape skins, making it more concentrated in the final product.

While moderate red wine consumption has been linked to potential health benefits, it is important to note that excessive alcohol consumption can have adverse effects on health, so moderation is key when considering red wine as a source of resveratrol.

Other Dietary Sources

In addition to red wine, there are several other dietary sources of resveratrol.

One of the most notable is grapes themselves, particularly red and purple varieties, which are rich in this polyphenol. Blueberries, cranberries, and certain other berries also contain resveratrol, though in smaller quantities.

Peanuts and pistachio nuts have been identified as good sources of resveratrol, along with the Japanese knotweed plant, which is considered one of the richest sources of this compound.

Cocoa and dark chocolate are additional sources of resveratrol, though they may contain lower levels compared to red wine and certain fruits.

Incorporating Resveratrol-Rich Foods
Incorporating resveratrol-rich foods into your diet can be a delicious and health-conscious choice.

Consuming red grapes as a snack or adding them to your salads and yogurt is a simple way to enjoy the potential benefits of resveratrol.

Berries, whether eaten fresh, frozen, or in smoothies, offer a flavorful and nutritious way to include resveratrol in your diet.

When it comes to nuts, snacking on peanuts and pistachios can be a satisfying way to introduce this compound into your meals. Additionally, dark chocolate can be a delightful treat for those looking to boost their resveratrol intake.

For those who are looking to obtain resveratrol without consuming alcohol or specific foods, resveratrol supplements are also available.

These supplements are often derived from Japanese knotweed and offer a convenient way to ensure a consistent intake of this polyphenol. However, it's important to consult with a healthcare professional before starting any supplementation regimen to ensure it aligns with your individual health goals and needs.

Resveratrol is a naturally occurring compound found in various foods and beverages, with red wine being one of the most well-known sources.

However, it can also be obtained from fruits, nuts, and even dark chocolate.

Incorporating resveratrol-rich foods into your diet can be an enjoyable way to potentially reap the health benefits associated with this polyphenol.

Additionally, for those who prefer not to rely on dietary sources, resveratrol supplements are available, although their use should be guided by professional advice to ensure safe and effective supplementation.

CHAPTER NINE

Resveratrol And Scientific Research

Resveratrol, a natural polyphenol found in various plants, including grapes, berries, and red wine, has garnered significant attention in the field of scientific research due to its potential health benefits.

This compound is known for its antioxidant properties and has been the subject of numerous studies aiming to explore its potential therapeutic applications.

Resveratrol is of particular interest because it is believed to play a role in the "French Paradox," which is the observation that despite a diet rich in saturated fats, the French population has a lower rate of heart disease. This paradox has been attributed to the moderate consumption of red wine and its resveratrol content.

Clinical Studies And Findings

Clinical studies on resveratrol have produced a wide range of findings, highlighting its potential effects on various aspects of human health. One of the most widely studied aspects of resveratrol is its role as an antioxidant.

Antioxidants are compounds that help protect cells from damage caused by free radicals, unstable molecules that can lead to oxidative stress and contribute to various diseases, including cancer, cardiovascular diseases, and neurodegenerative disorders.

Several studies have suggested that resveratrol's antioxidant properties may play a role in reducing the risk of these conditions.

Furthermore, resveratrol has been investigated for its potential anti-inflammatory properties. Chronic inflammation is a contributing factor to many chronic diseases, and resveratrol's ability to modulate inflammatory pathways has led to interest in its use as a therapeutic agent.

 Some studies have demonstrated that resveratrol can inhibit the activation of inflammatory markers and help reduce inflammation in various tissues.

Additionally, resveratrol has shown promise in the context of cardiovascular health. Research has indicated that resveratrol may have a positive impact on heart health by improving blood vessel function, reducing cholesterol levels, and preventing the formation of blood clots. These effects could potentially lower the risk of heart diseases, including heart attacks and strokes.

Cancer research has also explored the potential benefits of resveratrol.

While findings are not conclusive, some studies suggest that resveratrol might inhibit the growth of cancer cells and promote their apoptosis (cell death).

However, it's important to note that the anti-cancer effects of resveratrol are still being studied, and its efficacy as a cancer treatment remains uncertain.

Ongoing Research And Future Prospects

The research on resveratrol is ongoing, and there are several intriguing prospects for its future applications.

One of the challenges in studying resveratrol is its bioavailability, as it is rapidly metabolized and excreted from the body. Researchers are exploring various delivery systems and formulations to enhance its absorption and efficacy.

Resveratrol's potential role in longevity and age-related diseases is another area of ongoing investigation.

Some studies in animals, such as mice, have suggested that resveratrol might extend lifespan and improve metabolic health.

Whether these findings can be translated to humans remains a subject of continued research.

Another exciting avenue of exploration is resveratrol's impact on neurological health. Some studies have shown that resveratrol may have neuroprotective properties and could be beneficial in conditions like

Alzheimer's and Parkinson's disease. Further research is needed to understand the mechanisms involved and to develop potential therapies.

resveratrol has been a subject of intense scientific research due to its potential health benefits. It has shown promise in areas such as antioxidant activity, anti-inflammatory properties, cardiovascular health, and potential anti-cancer effects. Ongoing research is focused on improving its bioavailability, exploring its impact on longevity and age-related diseases, and investigating its potential in neurological health. While resveratrol holds promise, more research is needed to fully understand its mechanisms and therapeutic potential in various health conditions.

CHAPTER TEN

The Controversies And Myths

Resveratrol, a natural compound found in certain plants like grapes, has garnered significant attention in recent years for its potential health benefits.

However, with this attention, controversies and myths have also emerged. It's essential to examine these issues critically to gain a more accurate understanding of resveratrol and its role in human health.

Debunking Common Misconceptions

One of the most prevalent misconceptions surrounding resveratrol is its association with red wine.

While red wine does contain resveratrol, the concentration is relatively low. To obtain a therapeutic dose of resveratrol from wine, one would have to consume a substantial amount of alcohol, which can lead to more harm than good.

In contrast, resveratrol supplements provide a more controlled and potent source of the compound without the negative effects of excessive alcohol consumption.

Another misconception relates to the idea that resveratrol can replace a healthy diet and exercise regimen.

Some people believe that taking resveratrol supplements alone will lead to significant weight loss and improved cardiovascular health. In reality, resveratrol should be seen as a complementary component of a healthy lifestyle, not a standalone solution.

Its effects are more modest and work in conjunction with proper nutrition and regular physical activity.

Resveratrol's reputation as a miracle anti-aging compound is another common myth. While some studies have suggested potential anti-aging effects due to its antioxidant properties, it's important to recognize that aging is a complex process influenced by various factors.

Resveratrol may have a role in promoting cellular health, but it is not a fountain of youth. Individuals should maintain realistic expectations about the benefits of resveratrol.

Additionally, there is a misunderstanding that all resveratrol supplements are created equal. The quality and bioavailability of resveratrol supplements can vary significantly between brands and formulations.

Some products may not contain the claimed amount of resveratrol, while others may be in a form that is poorly absorbed by the body. It is crucial for consumers to do their research and choose reputable brands with transparent labeling to ensure they are getting the intended benefits.

Safety Concerns

Resveratrol is generally considered safe when taken in recommended doses, but safety concerns have been raised regarding high-dose supplementation.

Some studies have indicated that extremely high doses of resveratrol may have adverse effects on the liver and kidneys. These concerns highlight the importance of following dosing guidelines and consulting with a healthcare professional before taking high-dose supplements.

Another safety issue revolves around potential interactions with medications. Resveratrol may interact with certain drugs, such as blood thinners, and affect their effectiveness.

 It's crucial for individuals taking medications to consult with their healthcare provider before incorporating resveratrol supplements into their routine to avoid potential complications.

Pregnant and breastfeeding women should also exercise caution with resveratrol supplements, as there is limited research on its safety for these populations.

It is advisable to err on the side of caution and avoid unnecessary supplementation during these stages.

resveratrol is a fascinating compound with the potential for health benefits, but it is not a panacea.

Debunking common myths and understanding its limitations is essential for making informed decisions about its use. While it can be a valuable part of a health regimen when used correctly, safety concerns and misconceptions should be addressed to ensure its responsible and beneficial consumption.

CHAPTER ELEVEN

Resveratrol In Everyday Life:

Resveratrol, a natural polyphenol found in certain plants like grapes, red wine, and various berries, has gained considerable attention for its potential health benefits. This compound has been extensively studied for its antioxidant properties, which can help protect cells and tissues from oxidative stress and damage caused by free radicals.

The consumption of resveratrol has been associated with various health benefits, making it an interesting subject in the field of nutrition and wellness.

One of the most well-known sources of resveratrol is red wine, particularly in varieties like Pinot Noir and Cabernet Sauvignon.

Moderate red wine consumption, along with a balanced diet, is often considered a part of the Mediterranean diet, which has been linked to lower rates of heart disease and certain chronic conditions.

It's important to note that while resveratrol in red wine is often highlighted for its potential health benefits, the alcohol content in wine should be consumed in moderation.

Beyond red wine, resveratrol is also present in various foods, such as grapes, blueberries, raspberries, and peanuts.

These foods are not only delicious but also provide a natural source of resveratrol, making it easier to incorporate into your daily diet.

However, to fully harness the potential health benefits of resveratrol, some individuals turn to resveratrol supplements, which offer a more concentrated form of the compound.

Integrating Resveratrol Into Your Daily Routine:

Integrating resveratrol into your daily routine can be accomplished in several ways. One option is to consume resveratrol-rich foods regularly.

Grapes, for example, make for a healthy and delicious snack, and incorporating them into your daily diet can provide a steady source of resveratrol.

Berries like blueberries and raspberries can be added to breakfast cereals, yogurt, or smoothies. Nuts, particularly peanuts, can also be a part of your daily snacking routine.

For those who prefer the potential convenience and precise dosing that supplements offer, resveratrol supplements are available in various forms, including capsules and tablets.

When considering resveratrol supplementation, it's important to consult with a healthcare professional to determine the appropriate dosage for your individual needs. Additionally, be mindful of potential interactions with medications or existing health conditions.

Incorporating resveratrol into your daily routine can also involve cooking with ingredients that naturally contain this polyphenol.

Some recipes call for the use of red wine in cooking, and this can be a flavorful way to add resveratrol to your meals. However, it's important to remember that the alcohol in wine can evaporate during the cooking process, so not all of the resveratrol content may be retained.

Recipes And Meal Ideas:

Resveratrol can be incorporated into your diet through creative and delicious recipes. Here are a few meal ideas to inspire you:

Red Wine Reduction Sauce: Prepare a delicious red wine reduction sauce to accompany your favorite grilled meats or vegetables. Simmer red wine with shallots, garlic, and herbs to create a flavorful sauce that not only adds a touch of resveratrol but also enhances the taste of your dishes.

Resveratrol-Rich Smoothie: Create a resveratrol-rich smoothie by blending grapes, blueberries, and a splash of red wine for added flavor. You can sweeten it with honey or agave syrup and add yogurt for creaminess.

Mixed Berry Salad: Combine fresh raspberries and blueberries with a mix of greens, nuts, and feta cheese.

Drizzle with a red wine vinaigrette for a refreshing salad that provides both flavor and resveratrol.

Resveratrol-Infused Dessert: Try making a dessert like red wine-poached pears or berries with a red wine reduction. These treats not only taste exquisite but also offer the potential health benefits of resveratrol.

Incorporating resveratrol into your daily routine can be enjoyable and rewarding, whether you choose to do so through food sources, supplements, or creative cooking. Regardless of the method you prefer, it's essential to maintain a balanced and nutritious diet while considering your individual health needs and consulting with a healthcare professional if necessary.

Resveratrol is just one of many natural compounds that can contribute to a healthier lifestyle when used in moderation and as part of a well-rounded approach to wellness.

CHAPTER TWELVE

The Future Of Resveratrol

Resveratrol, a natural polyphenol found in various plants, such as grapes and red wine, has gained significant attention in recent years due to its potential health benefits. While its antioxidant properties have long been recognized, the future of resveratrol holds promising prospects in various domains.

This versatile compound has sparked interest in its emerging applications, potential breakthroughs, and the possibilities it presents for the fields of medicine and nutrition.

Emerging Applications

Resveratrol's emerging applications extend to diverse areas, including aging, cardiovascular health, neuroprotection, and even cancer prevention. In the context of aging, research suggests that resveratrol may activate sirtuins, a class of proteins linked to longevity and cellular health.

This activation could potentially slow down the aging process and reduce age-related diseases. Furthermore, resveratrol's ability to enhance endothelial function and reduce inflammation points to its potential for improving cardiovascular health.

Its role in neuroprotection is also fascinating, with studies indicating its ability to safeguard against neurodegenerative diseases like Alzheimer's and Parkinson's. These emerging applications offer hope for addressing major health concerns.

Potential Breakthroughs

In the world of science and medicine, resveratrol holds the promise of several potential breakthroughs. The compound's role in obesity management is of particular interest, as it has demonstrated the ability to activate brown adipose tissue (BAT), which can help in burning calories and regulating body weight.

Additionally, its anti-inflammatory and antioxidant properties may have implications in the management of chronic inflammatory conditions, such as arthritis and metabolic disorders.

Recent research also suggests that resveratrol might support bone health by stimulating osteoblasts, cells responsible for bone formation. These potential breakthroughs could revolutionize the way we approach obesity, inflammation, and bone-related issues.

Conclusion

the future of resveratrol is brimming with possibilities. This natural compound, found in various dietary sources, has garnered attention for its emerging applications in aging, cardiovascular health, and neuroprotection. Moreover, it holds the potential for breakthroughs in obesity management, chronic inflammation, and bone health. While extensive research is still required to fully understand the mechanisms and optimal dosage for these applications, resveratrol's journey from a dietary supplement to a promising candidate in various fields of science and medicine is a testament to the continuous exploration of nature's bounty for health and wellness. As we delve deeper into the intricacies of resveratrol, we may unlock its full potential and witness its transformative impact on human health and well-being.

www.ingramcontent.com/pod-product-compliance
Lightning Source LLC
Chambersburg PA
CBHW060753260726
48660CB00002B/604